T0157512

FITNESS, HEALTH & LONGEVITY

A Personal Journey

Frank Manganella

BALBOA.
PRESS

A DIVISION OF HAY HOUSE

Balboa Press books may be ordered through booksellers or by contacting:

Balboa Press
A Division of Hay House
1663 Liberty Drive
Bloomington, IN 47403
www.balboapress.com
1 (877) 407-4847

Because of the dynamic nature of the Internet, any web addresses or links contained in this book may have changed since publication and may no longer be valid. The views expressed in this work are solely those of the author and do not necessarily reflect the views of the publisher, and the publisher hereby disclaims any responsibility for them.

The author of this book does not dispense medical advice or prescribe the use of any technique as a form of treatment for physical, emotional, or medical problems without the advice of a physician, either directly or indirectly. The intent of the author is only to offer information of a general nature to help you in your quest for emotional and spiritual well-being. In the event you use any of the information in this book for yourself, which is your constitutional right, the author and the publisher assume no responsibility for your actions.

Any people depicted in stock imagery provided by Thinkstock are models, and such images are being used for illustrative purposes only.
Certain stock imagery © Thinkstock.

Print information available on the last page.

ISBN: 978-1-5043-6339-6 (sc)
ISBN: 978-1-5043-6340-2 (e)

Library of Congress Control Number: 2016912458

Balboa Press rev. date: 09/16/2016

CONTENTS

INTRODUCTION

This book is more than just an exercise manual. This book is different. Exercise is my passion. In fact, I am so passionate about exercise that I felt an overwhelming need to share with you my personal journey in discovering what I believe is the true meaning of exercise and incorporating the methods used by old-school strongmen of years gone by. They were the pioneers of strength, conditioning, fitness, and health. They were strong, healthy, fit, and flexible. They did not use supplements, steroids, diet pills, or caffeine-loaded drinks. In their prime, though, they could outperform any athlete today. What was their secret to strength, fitness, health, and longevity?

What started out as a personal journey to find the answer to that question led me to witness the most amazing transformations in myself and those I have had the privilege of training.

I feel the timing is perfect to write this book. We live in a fast-paced world where we expect and receive everything in an instant. There is instant banking, instant coffee, instant breakfast, and instant Internet, and we expect instant results from diet and exercise. Unfortunately, changes to the body occur slowly over time.

My goal is to convince you to slow down, introduce you to a (not-so-new but) different way of exercising, and share the physical and psychological results that I have witnessed with my clients, so you too can experience the numerous benefits that exercise and a healthy lifestyle have to offer.

Frank Manganella, NFPT certified professional trainer

PREFACE

"Exercise should be fun and enjoyable, it
should renew and invigorate you."

Jack LaLanne spoke those words on his TV show in the 1950s, and I remember them as though I heard them yesterday. For as long as I can remember, I have had a passion for muscle. Jack LaLanne, Steve Reeves, Charles Atlas, and Clint Walker were my boyhood idols. They had muscular physiques and were soft-spoken. I assumed that if you looked like they did, you really didn't have to say much. You just got respect. That belief was proven to me when I read the ads for the Charles Atlas Course in my favorite comic books. You know the ones. They showed the skinny guy with his girlfriend on the beach, but then the big muscle guy kicks sand in his face and walks away with the girl. The skinny guy purchases the course, does the exercises and his muscles are big. Back to the beach he goes to win back his girlfriend. That's impressive! Not only do you get respect, but you also get the girl. I purchased the course and felt that I was on my way to the perfect physique.

The course was full of illustrations on how to perform exercises. I knew there had to be more to it than just exercise. What did they eat? How much sleep did they get each night? How much water did they drink? What exactly did they do?

Many years later, still pondering that question, I happened to be in a bookstore and saw a magazine advertising a personal trainer certification course. I was so excited to find that advertisement. This was the first time I'd seen anything like it. At the time, the only course offered regarding exercise was to become a physical education teacher. As I looked at the ad, I thought, "Do I know as much as I think I know?" I had been lifting weights for fifteen years using muscle publications as my resource. I read everything at my disposal regarding exercise. I was yearning to learn more. Was I doing all the right things? I was hoping that this course would teach me how to look like my boyhood heroes. I purchased the course and studied the materials. At the time, the course was just what I was looking for. It explained how the body works regarding exercise, what exercises to perform based on a specific goal, and the importance of proper nutrition. I took the test and received my certification. It was official. On February 4, 1994, I became a certified personal trainer.

Little did I know that the journey I was about to undertake as a personal trainer would lead me to witness much, much more than just building muscle and developing the impressive physiques of my boyhood heroes.

CHAPTER 1

FITNESS—MY PERSONAL JOURNEY

Live Your Dream, and Dream Big

At the time I received my certification, I was employed as a sales representative. It was a great job with great pay and benefits. The only problem was that the company was going through a reduction in force. No one had job security. I was fortunate and had survived two company restructures. But late in 1994, while grocery shopping, I ran into an old friend I hadn't seen in a few years.

During our conversation, he asked if I was still lifting weights and whether I would be interested in training his son, a junior on his high school's cross country team. He expressed concern that the coaches wanted his son to get stronger but that he wasn't confident about their knowledge or ability regarding strength training. His son weighed only 103 pounds.

I responded that I would love to, informing my friend that I had just become certified basically to expand my personal knowledge. I learned to train with weights, not just lift them. I could do this in the basement of my home, where I had my own gym. I could train his son in the evening.

We started training on January 18, 1995. Our goal was to prepare him for a run that a local university was hosting in March. He trained diligently.

Late in the afternoon on the day of the big race, there was a knock at my door. It was my friend, glowing, with his son, my client, smiling like I'd never seen before. My client took his hands from behind his back and revealed his prize: a shiny trophy for a first-place finish. He had won the race. I was thrilled. He and his dad thanked me profusely, and my client said, "You know, there's something to this weight training. Do you think you can help my friend? He's on the basketball team and wants to get stronger."

I responded, "Absolutely!"

After planning the sessions and saying our good-byes, I closed my front door and experienced a feeling I never had before: a sense of accomplishment, pride, and joy. Just knowing that I might have had a positive impact on another's life moved me to tears. Now I had to know how many others I could help. I always had a dream about helping others in a big way. I was about to see.

One thing led to another, and within a short time, I had six high school student athletes training in my basement. It was amazing. The kids trained hard. I had the opportunity to listen to their complaints about high school sports, especially the lack of appreciation they felt from their coaches, parents, and fans. My basement became their safe place. There, they were able to train their bodies and clear their minds. They knew that I appreciated them and the effort they gave.

"This is so much bigger than just bending your arm with a weight in your hand," I thought. I was witnessing physical, mental, and spiritual changes in these young adults. Thus, I concluded that since we are body, mind, and spirit, once we begin to focus on one area of our being (in this case, the body), the other areas of our being start to speak up loud and clear. "Hey, I'm your spirit. I'm not happy. Help me too." The changes I'd witnessed in those young adults were bigger than big. They could only be described as miraculous. Their self-confidence grew, and they questioned and changed what was not working for them in their lives. They were strong, fit, and healthy.

Although they achieved what I described as miraculous results, I couldn't help but feel that there was a more efficient way to exercise. All of the lifting programs I researched and implemented with the student athletes called for either a two- or three-day split routine, which meant exercising some body parts on day one, other body parts on day two, and even other body parts on day three. Then, there is one day of rest, and you repeat the cycle. I felt that lifting so frequently was not necessary. Training my clients and myself in that manner didn't leave much time for anything else. The students were able to find time to study, but things like a social life or time for family were being compromised. The student athletes I trained did not have that kind of time or commitment to that type of training. I needed to prove my theory that the same miraculous results could be achieved without spending so many hours every day exercising.

A few years later, in 1997, I attended a Penn State football game. I was so impressed with the size, strength, speed, and flexibility of those athletes. Their physiques matched those of my boyhood heroes. I marveled at their pregame warm-up. They were executing drills with perfection. Suddenly, I heard someone blow a whistle on the field. The players jumped into single-file along on the field, five yards apart. Again, the whistle blew. Immediately, a hundred players went into a stretch position in unison and held it until the whistle blew again. They repeated this for several minutes, all in unison, no one out of step. What discipline! Who the hell was this man with the whistle? Searching the game program I had purchased, I discovered his name was John Thomas. He was the head strength-and-conditioning coach. "Wow! How the heck did they train? My athletes are good but not this good," I thought. When I returned home from the game, I immediately tried to find out how those athletes trained. I couldn't find any information. Damn!

Later that year, I attended a fitness seminar in Philadelphia sponsored by Reebok. I was so excited because I felt that the seminar would validate my intuition that training four, five, or six days a week was unnecessary and counterproductive and could possibly lead to injury. I had the opportunity to speak with some of the presenters and interact with many in attendance, but I left disappointed. I'm sure that if I had tested their body fat, it would have registered lean. I knew they had endurance just by my looking at them. Something was missing, though: They lacked that healthy glow. They just didn't look healthy. They were fit, but to me, they were not healthy.

My Search Ends

My excitement for Penn State football and my desire to learn more about the team's workouts led me to purchase season tickets. I couldn't help notice how much bigger, stronger, and faster the players got during their four or five years as a Penn State football player. The difference in physiques from freshman year to senior year was amazing. How the heck did they train?

December 27, 1999, is a day I will never forget, for it changed my life forever.

Penn State was playing Texas A&M in the Alamo Bowl in San Antonio, Texas, and I decided to attend the game. On the evening before the game, I was in the lobby of the hotel where the Penn State players and coaches were staying, and I saw John Thomas. I introduced myself, and we started talking about weight training and discovered that we shared many of the same philosophies regarding working out, supplements, and nutrition. We ended our conversation with JT (John Thomas) inviting me to attend his off-season winter workouts to see and learn firsthand the type of training done at Penn State. I had been invited to the Penn State weight room. Holy shit!

On January 15, 2000, another day I will never forget, JT, along with his assistant Jeremy Scott (who would later become the head strength-and-conditioning coach for football at Temple University), allowed me to witness firsthand what my intuition had been telling me all along.

I was blown away by how the athletes trained with weights. I'd never seen anything like it before—there was a total concentration and focus with a steady rhythm of sweat dripping off their foreheads. At Penn State, the athletes strength-trained their entire bodies in one hour. Since the human body functions as one unit, total body training is the logical approach.

I finally found the healthy glow I was searching for in the faces and body language of the athletes at Penn State. Yes, they were young men in their prime, but so too had been the participants at the seminar I had attended in Philadelphia a year earlier.

The athletes at Penn State just looked fit and healthy. They were strong, flexible, and in incredible condition, just like my boyhood heroes, the old-school strongmen. As I learned more about the training at Penn State, I discovered the following key points:

- Based on the sport season, they lifted two or three times per week for one-hour sessions. Many people today overestimate how much time they have to dedicate to exercise to live a long, healthy life.
- In those one-hour sessions, they worked hard. There was no bullshit—it was work or go home. Based on my experience, one hour was not a lot of time to work out; it was the quality of the workout that mattered, not the quantity of time or quantity of exercises.
- In those one-hour sessions, they did exercises for their entire body, usually performing only one set of an exercise. This was not the norm. Everything I knew up to that point was doing multiple sets, usually three, of every exercise ever invented for a body part. Those athletes knew how to achieve the effect of multiple sets in just one set. This was mind-blowing. Later, I discovered that in the mid-1940s, Dr. Thomas Delmore used multiple sets in rehabilitating World War II veterans. This is the protocol for lifting weights even to this day.
- They did aerobic training on the days when they were not lifting.
- Both male and female athletes performed this type of training.

The name of this training is HIT, high-intensity training, developed by Arthur Jones in the 1970s.

I immediately knew the HIT strength-training program would be a perfect fit for my clients. They would have the option of training two or three times a week for one-hour sessions. We would do one set of an exercise for every body part, training the entire body in one session. The only thing they had to learn was how to lift hard and execute the perfect rep every time.

It was pure and simple with no frills or gimmicks—just working your muscles hard in a slow manner using proper form until positive muscle failure (which means you cannot do another rep without momentum, swinging, or jerking).

Buddha once said, "Do not believe in anything simply because you have heard it. Do not believe in anything simply because it is spoken and rumored by many or it is found written in your religious books. Do not believe in traditions because they have been handed down for many generations. But after observation and analysis, when you find that anything agrees with reason and is conducive to the good and benefit of one and all, then accept it and live up to it."

This form of weight training just feels right to me. After observation and analysis, HIT falls in line with my beliefs and is conductive to the good and benefit of one and all.

Once again, the basic element of this strength-training system is to perform every repetition in every set in a slow, controlled motion to minimize momentum and maximize muscle tension and fiber recruitment.

I couldn't wait to implement this training method with my clients, especially with my student athletes and younger clients.

CHAPTER 2

HEALTH—MY PERSONAL JOURNEY

While all this was happening in my basement, I was still working in sales, but I was becoming less and less interested in it. I was being so fulfilled training the student athletes that the dog-eat-dog world of sales was wearing me down.

Once again, my body, mind, and spirit were aligned, but my mind and spirit were saying, "Hey, this sales job is killing you." Of course, I didn't listen and continued doing both jobs until I had an eye-opening experience.

I knew deep down that the sales job was becoming more and more stressful. The downsizing continued. People were losing their jobs. I kept getting staffed, but there were with larger sales territories and some overnight trips. With those changes, I had to sacrifice my time training the students. I was now training twelve kids. Both jobs were being compromised. I was not happy, nor was I raised to believe in doing a half-assed job. Oh, how I prayed for an answer.

Looking back, I know now that the universe, God, destiny—whatever title you choose to call it—was sending me the signs I was praying for. The problem was that I was so preoccupied with prayer that I failed to recognize the signs that I was receiving.

One day, while scanning the television stations, I stopped at a channel that was broadcasting a speech by Les Brown, a very famous motivational speaker. His message was that there is greatness inside you and that you should not to die with your dreams, desires, and ideas unfulfilled. This left me breathless and inspired. Still, I prayed for an answer. During Sunday Mass, I listened attentively to a sermon about a CEO who decided to leave corporate America and pursue his dream to be a teacher. He taught in one of the poorest and most violent school districts in New York. He was directly responsible for a countless number of his students becoming successful. Sadly, he was shot, killed, and robbed by one of the students in the district. The moral was that if you put your hand on someone's shoulder and that person walks away with your imprint, you have succeeded in life. What a message! Once again, I was left breathless and inspired. Still, I continued to pray.

Late one Friday, after one of the most stressful days on the sales job, I decided to go for a jog to clear my head, calm my thoughts, and figure out how to handle the pressure I was feeling from training the students and performing the sales job. During my run, it happened. I felt enormous pressure and tightness in my chest, I had difficulty breathing, and I was sweating profusely. "Holy shit! I'm having a heart attack," I said to myself. "F**k! This is the big one. Damn, I'm only forty years old, and I know I'm in good shape. What the f**k?" Somehow, I made it home.

I must have been in a state of denial because I waited until the following Monday to call my doctor and explain what had happened. He ordered me to the hospital, and I was given a stress test. Shortly after the test, during which I tried my hardest to imitate the feelings I had had on the jog, my doctor came in, looked me in the eye, and said, "Frank, you're fine. You're the healthiest guy I know, and the results of your stress test prove that. I'm sure you know that negative expectations, fear, and anxiety can actually make people feel ill. Are you under stress?"

I replied, "Yes, a tremendous amount. But this was real! Do your mean to tell me that my mind can have this effect on my body?"

"Yes, absolutely," he said. I recall an example of this phenomenon. You imagine cutting a lemon in half, put it into your mouth, and bite down on it. Notice that your mouth produced more saliva. That is the power of the mind. My doctor continued, "Let me prescribe something for you." Now, I'm not a fan of pills. I know many people who think they are great and rely on them to function, they are not for me.

I recall a quote that read, "You can tell a person's health by how many he takes two of—pills or stairs."

I'm more of a prevention kind of guy, not someone who just wants my symptoms treated. There is an old aphorism that reads, "Prevention is better than cure." I knew the source of my stress, and I also knew that there are two ways to handle stress—accept it (cope) or make a change (run like hell). I thanked my doctor and went home to try to figure out what to do with my life. Should I start taking medication? I didn't want chemicals in my body. When I arrived home, my decision became clear. Waiting for me was a certified letter from my employer stating that another downsizing was on the way. I was staffed, but I was to have a larger sales territory and even more overnight stays. My new assignment meant that I would leave my house on Monday morning and come home Friday night.

"Oh no," I thought. "What about the kids?" I refused the new assignment, resigned from my sales job, and put my heart and soul into training those student athletes. Prayer answered!

The lesson I learned was that life as we know it can change in an instant. Feeling like I was having a heart attack made me realize how precious life is. I recall watching Oprah Winfrey one afternoon way back in 1995. Her first guest was someone who invented a digital clock that was designed to run backward. In fact, I saw one in my local post office in 1999 counting down to the millennium. As this digital clock was running backward, Oprah asked her guest, "So why did you invent this?"

He responded, "Well, let's say you're pregnant. You can program nine months in hours and minutes and time the birth of your baby. Or, let's say you're getting married. You can program the number of hours and minutes until your wedding day."

Oprah then responded, "Wow, three minutes of my life just went by!"

"Yes," he said. "I really didn't design it to do that, but you can also program seventy-eight years of life expectancy and watch the time tick away."

They went to a commercial break, and the show returned with another guest whose expertise was how to get the most out of the short time you're here. Several principles were discussed, but one just hit me like a ton of bricks. It read: "If an opportunity presents itself to you, and you view that opportunity as a deathbed regret, you should pursue it."

I was presented with an opportunity to change lives and be who I am—actually, who we all are: love and kindness. Goodbye, sales, and hello, personal training.

It was time to put my knowledge and education into action. Since I committed to train full-time, I made a personal vow to create an atmosphere where my clients could actually look forward to exercising, have fun doing it, and continue to exercise their entire life. That would be my legacy. That would be my contribution to society. If I could achieve that, I would have done my job.

Middle Age

Life changes at middle age. It sure did for me. I resigned from a job that was killing me to peruse my dream. Even with my lifestyle, I felt my body change. I felt myself gaining a few extra pounds, and I discovered that shedding those extra pounds was not as easy as it was when I was younger. This is a time of life when many become less active. You work long hours with long commutes, you may be raising children, and leisure time is a thing of the past. Your health begins to feel the effects of this hectic, stressful, and sedentary lifestyle. Many begin medications or are advised by their doctor to start exercising. Once again, the HIT method is ideal for those who are middle age. With HIT training, you can work out two or three times per week for one hour each session, thus leaving plenty of time for work, family, and life. Plus, if you are like the many people who don't enjoy exercise to begin with, HIT training makes perfect sense because it takes less time than other programs. Results from a 2016 *Parade Magazine*/Cleveland Clinic survey found that the biggest barrier to physical activity was a lack of time. All I'm asking for is two hours a week. It is a small investment for big benefits.

Here are the facts: There is scientific evidence that strength training (also known as resistance training) boosts metabolism. You keep burning fat for up to two days afterward. Aerobic exercise does not. Resistance training can tone and strengthen muscles for any person. It can be done with lightweight rubber tubing, weights, or weight machines. Notice I use the term "training." There is a big difference between weight training and weightlifting.

Weight training increases serotonin output. Serotonin is responsible for sleep, mood, and appetite. Researchers have found that heavy weight training releases endorphins, which alleviate anxiety and depression and act as a painkiller. Studies also show that exercise works as well as prescription medicine for some people suffering chronic anxiety.

Students and Young Adults

The primary focus when training young people is to develop their coordination and to enhance their self-esteem. I cannot begin to tell you how successful I have been achieving this using the HIT method. Watching these young people discover the physical strength and mental power we all possess is breathtaking.

They all start out the same way: easily distracted, unsure of themselves, a little clumsy (due to their ever-changing and developing bodies), and even a little frightened. But once the training starts and they learn how to perform exercise after exercise slowly and in proper form, distractions disappear, confidence builds, coordination improves, and strength grows, and they experience a sense of achievement. They learn how to leave their comfort zone and that taking a risk will not kill them. These are two priceless life lessons.

The Big Four

I've trained elementary, high school, and college students; males and females; people of all ages (even in their eighties); and people fighting the effects of Lyme disease, thyroid issues, low back pain, and even cancer. They all had four things in common: attitude, determination, commitment, and consistency.

Attitude

The transformation I've witness with all my clients is miraculous to say the least. Weakness is replaced with strength, shyness and uncertainty with confidence, illness with improved health. There is better balance and improvements in body weight and composition. My seniors became agile not fragile. The people I had the honor of training came to me for a variety of reasons. They all possess a positive attitude. Attitude is everything.

Determination

Along with a positive attitude, they were determined to change what wasn't working in their lives. Nothing gets in the way of their workouts. Vacation, travel, job commitments, rain, snow, sleet, and even the common cold can't stop them. Yes, some had occasional setbacks, but they never stopped working out. One client continued training even when dealing with adverse effects of chemotherapy treatment. What a role model!

Commitment

Exercise is a lifelong commitment. It is especially important to exercise as you age. Once my clients made the commitment to work out, it was my job to implement the words of the great Jack LaLanne. I must find a way to make this fun and enjoyable, and I know this will renew and invigorate them. If I can achieve that, they will be consistent. It was easy for me to do so using the HIT method. My clients are excited about the fact that they don't have to exercise every day for hours and hours and are never bored with their workouts. And this is despite the fact that I never change the exercises they do. I occasionally change the order of the exercises or the cadence of the lifting, and by doing that, every workout is a new experience. Once they learn the exercise and the ability to perform the perfect repetition, results are almost immediate.

Consistency

My experience has been that my clients who were consistent with their workouts made the most improvements and achieved the best results. The key to long-lasting health is consistency.

When I was young, my mother would constantly tell me to brush my teeth. I was reminded over and over again that once my second set of teeth came in, they were the last set I was ever going to get. To maintain them and keep them healthy, my mother made sure I brushed them at least twice a day. No one ever preached to me that this is the only body I am going to get. No one stressed the importance of exercising the body, feeding it nutritious food, giving it proper rest, respecting it, and appreciating it for all the miraculous processes it does without any effort on my part. I never have to think about my heart beating, my kidneys and liver functioning, or it healing me when I catch the common cold. It just does it every day.

Exercise your body as consistently as you brush your teeth.

CHAPTER 3

LONGEVITY—MY PERSONAL JOURNEY

The Magic Pill

I've been a personal trainer now for over twenty years. I have exercised since I can remember. I owned and operated my own gym and had the good fortune of being appointed a strength and conditioning coach at my local high school. I can definitely write a book (like this one) on the many exercises that have come and gone; the latest supplement developed to make you big and strong; and what exactly is the magic pill to make boys stronger and muscles bigger, girls to be fit and feminine, and seniors to continue to be active and energetic.

It took a few tragedies in my life to find my magic pill. My grandfather developed pancreatic cancer. As I researched his illness, (something I always do since I'm big on preventing not treating illness), I discovered that one of the things you can do to prevent such a tragedy is exercise. A few years later, without any warning, my father was rushed to the hospital where they performed emergency surgery on both his carotid arteries. Once again, I was curious as to how to prevent this, and once again, one of the things you can do is exercise. My mother had hypertension, as did other members of her family. Hoping that this was not in my future, I decided to investigate how I could prevent this from happening to me. Exercise. As I began to read about disease prevention, a common theme kept appearing. Whether I was researching heart disease, hypertension, cancer, or even preventing the common cold, the one constant was exercise. Exercise is the magic pill.

And why not? It makes total sense. We have the same bodies as our ancestor the caveman. We are designed with fingers and toes for a reason—to hunt and gather. Our bodies were meant to move. Sitting in front of computers and television sets for hours and hours is killing us. We were meant to move. Since we don't hunt or gather anymore, we must exercise. We were meant to move. (I'm repeating this for a reason.)

One hundred and fifty years ago, a person was lucky to live past age fifty. Thanks to the inventions of sanitation, vaccination, and medication, our lives have extended. Today, our life expectancy is around seventy-eight years, and we should make darn sure we're healthy enough to enjoy a high quality of life.

I remember listening to Dr. Deepak Chopra define cancer as a cell that lost its memory. My interpretation of his definition is as follows: Every cell in our body has two functions, to decay and rebuild. If you are exercising, the cell dies and is replaced with a stronger cell. That cell dies, and another strong cell replaces it. Now, if you are sedentary, your cell dies, and a weaker cell replaces it. It dies, and another weaker cell is formed. This continues until a cell is formed that no longer knows what it is supposed to do. All of your cells are in a constant state of renewal. You choose if those new cells come in strong or weak.

A few years ago, I was searching for a used car for my son. One afternoon, parked in the lot of a small produce market, was a car with a for-sale-by-owner sign in the front window. I went into the market and inquired as to who was selling the car. I discovered that it belonged to the mother of a gentleman in his sixties, who was a friend of the owner. It was like hitting the lottery, a car driven by a little old lady. Mint condition with low mileage.

I met with the owner's son, took the car for a test drive, and negotiated a fair price. The only thing left to do was have the title of the car registered in my name. We agreed that I would come to his home later that day to get the paperwork and complete the transaction. When I arrived at his home, he invited me to have a seat in his kitchen where he introduced me to his wife. "I want you to meet my mother too," he said. He left the kitchen, went down a hall, and returned with his mother. She was in her eighties, bent at the waist, and walked with his assistance. "Mom, I'd like you to meet Frank," he said. I stood up, approached her, and extended my hand to greet her.

She said to me, "They told me I can't drive anymore. Are you taking my car away from me?"

My heart sank into my stomach. I saw the defeat in her teary eyes. Her independence was gone. Although her mind was sharp and her vision was great (with the help of glasses), she could no longer stand up straight or get up out of a chair. She was frail and could no longer drive her car due to her loss of mobility.

This was a prime example of weak cells being replaced with weaker cells.

I can't begin to imagine what I would do if someone made the decision that I didn't have the ability to drive my own car. I couldn't help but think that this must be the kiss of death.

I assured her that I would take care of her car. I promised that I would wash and wax it and told her how much I appreciated her taking such good care of it. I also made a vow to myself that I would do everything in my power to prevent that scenario from happening to me. How can I prevent myself from becoming frail as I get older? How can I make sure that my cells are strong? Exercise, weight training in particular. Since gravity is constantly pushing down on us, we must have a strong muscular system to keep us upright against this constant force and to prevent osteoporosis.

I want you to imagine the human skeleton. Without muscle, it would be a pile of bones on the ground. Without a strong muscular system to hold us up against the force of gravity, we will bend at the waist and need assistance to move.

During the writing of this book, I witnessed another event to validate my belief that exercise is the magic pill. On a beautiful sunny Sunday morning, I received a phone call from one of my clients notifying me that she had to admit her husband, age eighty-four, into an assisted living facility. He had suffered a stroke a few years earlier. Sadly, the stroke impaired his vision and memory. His wife was a marvelous caretaker, but that responsibility was taking its toll on her health and well-being. After meeting with family members, they all agreed that he would receive excellent care in the facility, and it would be the best option for both of them. I spent the afternoon with them at the facility. The facility was beautiful. The staff was friendly and caring. There were many activities to give the residents an active social life. The food was delicious. I couldn't help but think, "Thank God there are places like this to care for our elderly."

Still, I felt uneasy. Most of the residents walked with the aid of walkers or canes and were bent over at the waist. "What if they did exercises for their core when they were younger?" I thought. "What if they began training with weights now? Would they still be bent over?"

After spending a few hours with them, I sat in my car and promised myself that I would do everything in my power to try to avoid that same fate. Exercise hard, eat right, and get plenty of sleep, eliminate or handle stress. I must do the things I must do and without exception.

In both stories, the people I saw bent over at the waist could have been experiencing sarcopenia along with other factors associated with aging. Sarcopenia is a medical term for muscle loss that becomes relatively severe. Sarcopenia's effects can include decreased muscle strength, mobility issues, weak bones, diabetes, a loss of physical function, and more. Many of us will lose muscle as we age. On average, this occurs at a rate of one to two percent a year between the ages thirty and fifty years and about three percent between age fifty and seventy years. Our arms and legs weaken, looking thin or flabby. It becomes harder to execute everyday tasks. We then become less active, frail, have our car taken from us, wind up in assisted living, and may even develop chronic disease.

Many studies have shown that older people who do resistance training can significantly improve their muscle strength and performance, even after just a couple of months of training. Any strength training can help prevent or treat sarcopenia, but research has shown that strenuous workouts are most effective.

Along with strength training, it's equally beneficial to perform exercises for your core. The core muscles are located between your pelvis and the area just under your breastbone, in both the front and back. They are the deepest abdominal muscle (transversus abdominis), which is responsible for supporting the lumbar spine, and the deepest back muscle (multifidus) as well as other muscles such as the internal obliques. The pelvic floor also works with the deep abdominal muscles. To feel the core muscles in action, place your hand on your belly button and cough. You will feel your midsection brace and tighten deep in your body as if you are wearing a corset or belt around your spine. When you train and strengthen your core muscles, your spine is supported, you are less vulnerable to injury, and your balance improves. Exercises to strengthen trunk or core muscles also increase spinal bone density for women, thereby protecting them from osteoporosis. There are two types of exercises that are important for building and maintaining bone density: weight-bearing and muscle-strengthening exercises. Now we have the fate and future of the American athlete. No longer are we the average American.

One cold, wintry evening, as I was leaving my gym and walking to my car, my core muscles were challenged. A fresh blanket of snow had just fallen, covering the ground, sidewalk, and my car. It also covered a patch of ice on the ground a short distance from my car, making it invisible. When I walked on the snow covered patch of ice, both feet slipped out from underneath me. I was falling. My body was horizontal, and I felt like I was falling in slow motion. I felt my core muscles brace (just like they do when I cough), and I felt my glutes (butt muscles) tighten (to protect my tail bone). I hit the ground with a thud.

As I sat in the fresh snow, I began to assess the damage. I felt fine. Nothing broken! I chuckled, and that little voice inside me remarked, "Strong core!"

I have clients who have had the same experience when they sustained a fall. They all told me that the fall was in slow motion and that nothing broke.

CHAPTER 4

HIGH-INTENSITY TRAINING

The Perfect Rep: The White-Light Method

In the world of exercise, the term "rep" is used frequently. It is short for repetition. A repetition is one complete movement of a particular exercise. It is a means to count the number of exercise movements.

When I was young, I used to enjoy watching *Wide World of Sports* and the Olympics on television. Olympic weightlifting was one of my favorites. The weightlifter executes a lift with an enormous amount of weight for one rep. His lift was immediately determined by judges and referees as to whether it was a successful lift. The lift had to be perfect. Usually, the judges' and referees' results were registered via a lighting system with a white light indicating a successful lift and a red light indicating a failed lift.

Slow Power: Quality vs Quantity

I inform my clients that in order to get my white light, they have to execute a perfect rep every time. It has to be slow on the lowering and slow on the lifting, with a pause in the middle, usually in a four, two, four cadence. You lower the weight for a four count, pause for a two count, lift the weight for a four count, and repeat. I adjust the resistance for my clients to achieve the repetition range I am expecting from them.

They have to execute each rep in its full range of motion. At times, I vary the cadence to a two, one, three, but regardless of the cadence I use, my emphasis is to always have the client follow the following HIT principles:

- Use proper form
- Have a high level of intensity
- Push yourself as hard as you can to improve each time
- Work to success, which means you cannot possibly do one more rep without compromising form.

To achieve the principles mentioned above, one very important thing has to happen. We must take a risk and leave our comfort zone. We all have a comfort zone. The moment we feel the effects of exercising our muscles, our heart rate increases and our breathing becomes rapid. We stop, and we hit our comfort zone. It's time to take a risk. A lot of people think sweating and being winded are bad signs. They think it means they can't handle exercise. Instead, think of sweat as evidence of progress. You're doing something that is good for your body. All that hard breathing and sweat is helping you achieve your fitness goals. We must dare to leave our comfort zone and discover new possibilities.

Intensity

The word "intensity" is used so frequently today. It's used to describe workout programs and is spoken to clients by trainers as motivation. Many times, I hear trainers telling their clients to keep things intense.

To me, the proper term is "intensity of effort". Somewhere along the way, "of effort" disappeared. Intensity took its place. As a personal trainer, my job is to get you to work as hard as you possibly can for every rep and every set (a set is several repetitions intended to be done in series).

We all possess the ability to perform incredible feats of strength under the right circumstances. If you witness a car run over an infant, you will lift that car. The strength potential of the human body is remarkable. There is documentation of people surviving events that should have killed them. I try to get my clients to tap into that potential. Lift with maximum effort using proper form without cheating, jerking, straining, or momentum—for just one set.

One Set to Success—Time Under Load

Many people lifting weights worry too much about how much weight they are using and not nearly enough about how well they are doing lifting it. Many just run through a set of reps. One hard set done in proper form is far better than sets just done. Each set and each rep of each set should be done hard so that you get the very most out of it.

I am blessed to have a client whose passion is physics. He understands the importance of slow movements. He has shared the definition of action. Action is force times distance times time.

If we increase the time, action will increase along with it, causing more work on the muscle. Our muscles respond to work. If we apply the science of physics to our workouts, the HIT method makes total sense. Always think about time under load. The more time the muscle is working, the better the results will be.

Cardiovascular Training—Sprinting

Studies validate the fact that the human body was not designed to run marathons. Rather, it was meant to sprint short distances. Research also discovered that even though we burn fat when we jog at sixty to seventy percent of our maximum heart rate, the human body, in its infinite intelligence, stores more fat, thus having the reverse effect we are striving for. Even animals in the wild never jog. When it is hungry, it will run as fast as it can (sprint) until it catches its prey. If it can't catch it, it will stop, recover, and sprint after another. If you have ever been told by your doctor to take a stress test, you will be required to get your heart rate to eighty-five percent of maximum. Once at eight-five percent, you stop. The time it takes to get your heart rate down to sixty percent of maximum is recorded and reveals your state of health.

I have three rules of thumb when sprinting.

One: Regardless of how long you sprint, your rest time in between sprints should double the time sprinting. For example, if you sprint for fifteen seconds, rest for thirty seconds before the next sprint.

Two: Keep your work time (sprinting) to ten minutes total and the elapsed time to around thirty minutes. For example, one minute warming up, one minute sprinting, and resting two minutes between sprints. Repeat this ten times. The result is ten minutes of sprinting with an elapsed time of twenty-nine minutes.

Three: Keep your heart rate to eighty-five percent of maximum. I use the following formula: 220 − your age = maximum heart rate. If you are fifty years old, the formula would read 220 − 50 = 170. Your maximum heart rate is 170 beats per minute. Eighty-five percent of 170 is 144.5 beats per minute.

If you are in good condition, you can get your heart rate up to ninety percent, but be sure to exit that zone quickly. Your body will start to feed on muscle for energy when exercising at a heart rate of eighty-six percent or higher. You've worked too damn hard in your weight training workouts to lose the muscle you are building.

CHAPTER 5

PHYSICAL CHANGES—MORE THAN MUSCLE

Illness or Injury Recovery

My experience has been that there is a direct correlation between how fit you are and how healthy you are. To me, fit means strong, sound, and energetic. Healthy is free of disease. My clients and I are rarely ill, but when an occasional illness does enter our lives, we recover quickly.

I believe the reason for quick recovery and healing is this: When you exercise, you break down muscle fibers. Immediately after exercise, your body goes into repair. Since we repeat this day after day, week after week, month after month, our bodies are healing machines. Our bodies become very efficient at healing. So if there ever is a trauma to our bodies, we heal quickly. I had the opportunity to test this theory.

Many years ago, when I was a freshman in high school, I was on the basketball team. During a practice in January 1969, I took a nasty fall, which resulted in a compound fracture in my right leg. It required surgery to set the bones back in place. Long story short, I healed nicely, resumed playing sports, and never had any issues with the leg. However, I always had weakness and soreness in my left shoulder as a result of the fall. Over time, the pain got worse and worse, especially when I would reach overhead, something I had to do many times a day as a trainer. In 2014, the pain was so severe and my range of motion was so limited that I had developed lower back pain. I was twisting my body to lift my arm. I was protecting the arm so much that I strained to train a client. Immediately, I knew I had strained so badly that I caused an inguinal hernia.

My biggest fear was the MRI. There was no way was I going into that damn thing. Well, I had to get way out of my comfort zone because the doctor required an MRI to determine my injury. Again, because I was raised to believe in never doing anything in a half-assed fashion, the MRI revealed that I no longer had cartilage in my shoulder joint. It was bone on bone, and the only procedure to alleviate my pain and return my range of motion was total joint replacement surgery. I firmly believe that because my muscles were strong, it took forty-five years before I had to take action on the injury I sustained in high school. My mission was to put a plan into action for life after surgery.

First, I wanted to be in the best physical shape of my life. Second, I needed to have the surgery, which required six weeks in a sling and four months of therapy. Third, I had to get the shoulder as strong as possible. That meant that while the repaired arm was healing in a sling, I had to continue to exercise the nonsurgically repaired arm and all my other body parts. The human body functions as one unit. There are many studies validating how much faster athletes recover from surgery when they continue to train. Fourth: Have the hernia surgically repaired.

I can honestly say that I achieved all my goals. As a result of my plan, I was out of the sling and into therapy within five weeks. I required only three months of therapy and had excellent results with the inguinal hernia surgery as well. I even had my one-year follow-up doctor visit for my shoulder in fifty weeks, two weeks early. This was proof to me that my body knows how to repair and rebuild cells quickly and efficiently. It's true—the better physical shape you are in, the better you heal.

My clients who have experienced physical trauma in their lives have experienced similar, amazing results. One client had a surgical procedure performed by a cardiologist and was scheduled for monthly follow-up visits. After seven months of HIT training, her cardiologist gave her a big smile, told her how proud he was of her, and reduced her visits to every other month. The better physical shape you are in, the better you heal.

Use of Medications

Many of my clients have to take prescription medication. Regardless of the reason for needing the medication, they all have had positive results from exercise.

My clients who take medication due to genetics have been able to maintain their dose without any increases for many years. This is just another benefit of exercise.

I have a difficult time putting into words how this makes me feel. Happy, elated, thrilled, excited, moved—I just can't describe the emotion when you know you have had a positive impact on someone's life. This is so much bigger than me showing you how to bend your arm with a weight in hand. There are many different reasons why my clients began exercising with me. Weight loss, toning, and strength are just a few. When we begin, I become an instructor in the proper execution of an exercise. Over time, I become therapist, sounding board, stress reliever, comedian, role model, and confidant. I love my job.

CHAPTER 6

THE ULTIMATE PSYCHOLOGICAL BENEFIT

Up to this point, my focus was to explain the physical benefits of exercise. Now, I want to share with you my main motivation for writing this book. My goal for you is to experience quieting the mind.

One of my client, the physicist I mentioned earlier, described his experience with HIT training as follows: "The great thing about this is it gets you to a pure state."

When you train the way I am describing, you take your thoughts away from your everyday life events and actually experience the benefits of meditation. I learned that the object of meditation is quieting the mind to hear your soul, spirit, and intuition—whatever you wish to call it. With practice and by implementing various techniques such as focusing on normal breathing or the sound of the ocean, you can stop the chatter. You can actually become in tune with your soul, intuition, and spirit.

When you lift weights slowly, you cannot help but to focus on the working muscle. The mind becomes quiet, and you achieve the benefits of meditation. You enter the pure state my client referred to. This is one of the reasons that you start to hear the other areas of your being, mind and spirit, loud and clear.

This is when I witness clients making profound changes in their lives.

The young athletes just knew that they were physically stronger and mentally tougher than their opponent but were gentle enough to lend a helping hand when their opponent was knocked down.

Those in their middle age years began questioning some of the choices they made earlier in their lives and found the courage to change what wasn't working. They were being guided by intuition, spirit, or whatever you choose to call it.

The corporate executives dealing with stress and work-related issues experienced clarity in their decision-making.

My discovery was that we have the answers to whatever we are seeking already inside us. All we have to do is silence the thinking mind.

CHAPTER 7

NUTRITION AND WEIGHT MANAGEMENT

"Be sure to finish your dinner. Don't waste food. There are people starving in some far away country."

"You can't go out and play until you finish your meal."

These words of wisdom and threats my mother would tell me when I was a young boy.

One day, I couldn't take it anymore and responded, "Geez, Mom, I can't eat anymore. I'm full. If those people are starving, let's send them some food." I quickly learned that disrespect was another reason I couldn't go out and play with my friends.

We learn to overconsume at a very young age. I believe it's as early as when we are able to eat baby food. Mom is spoon feeding us. Since we can't verbally tell her that we have had enough, we begin spitting out the food, only to have mom wipe our chin with the spoon and shove it back into our mouths. Our little brain starts to process this event and develops the conclusion that we don't know what's good for us. Rather, the big people do. We surrender our intuition to others.

Parents and even religion dictate to us how much as well as when and what we eat. The good thing is that our intuition did not leave us.

We know when we are hungry, and we know when we are full. The bad thing is that in today's fast-paced world, weight management is not as easy as food in (energy in) and food out (energy out).

Today, food is not only used for energy. It is also used for comfort, stress relief, and celebration. It's estimated that obesity is associated with

28

ten to twenty-five percent of all deaths and shortens life expectancy by four to seven years. Sadly, our modern society promotes obesity because we have easy access to high calorie foods and have jobs that allow us to avoid physical activity.

Shortly after I began exercising and really listening to my intuition, I discovered that I was overeating because of the message I kept hearing as a young boy. I needed to prove to my mother, who is deceased, that I'm a good boy. I'm not disrespectful, and I want to go out and play. I realized that my mother was giving me this advice for a reason. She heard it from her parents when she was a little girl too. I now realize why leftovers were such a bad thing when my mom was a young girl. Her parents were Italian immigrants and had little income. Refrigeration was not yet invented, so there were only two options when it came to meals—finish your plate or throw it out for the birds (thus wasting food and the hard-earned money used to purchase the ingredients).

Today, we are blessed with refrigerators, ovens, and microwaves. We have the ability to prepare large quantities of food, eat enough to satisfy our hunger, and then refrigerate the leftovers for another meal. Therefore, all you have to do is eat your meal and walk away when your hunger is satisfied.

It sounds so easy, but the reality is that it takes will power, determination, and effort. I remember when I decided to stop when I was full. I was sitting with a tray of pizza before me. There were eight slices of the most delicious pizza I ever had. "What a lousy time to do this," I thought. In the past, I would have eaten those eight slices without even blinking, I placed the tray on the counter behind me, took one slice from the box, placed it on my plate, and ate it slowly, enjoying every bite. When I finished that slice, I paused and asked myself whether I was still hungry. The answer was that I wasn't. I was full after one slice of pizza when I used to eat the whole thing. I refrigerated the remaining slices and ate them later. I was amazed at how little food satisfied my hunger.

I believe we have to identify other factors in our lives that may be causing us to overconsume food. According to research, some of the factors of overeating, thus resulting in weight gain are:

Stress
Lack of sleep
Not drinking enough water
Poor digestion
Not eating enough fiber
Hormonal or glandular issues
Vitamin deficiency
Excess alcohol
Prescription drugs
Emotions (depressed, upset, angry, lonely, happy, excited)
Severe calorie cutbacks
High-octane exercise drills
I feel that there is another reason for overeating and weight gain.
As human beings, we don't do anything that doesn't serve us.

The smokers who say they want to quit, yet continue to smoke, are benefitting from smoking. Someone who says that their weight loss efforts are in vain could be hording the excess weight because it serves them. It's almost like self-sabotage. When I have a client who is struggling with losing weight, using love and kindness, I have a heart-to-heart conversation with the client.

What works best for me is asking my client to finish my sentence. Their answer must be immediate and without thinking.

My sentence: "Weight loss is?" Or "When I lose weight?" The answers are their deep beliefs regarding weight loss.

Some examples of answers are:

Weight loss is: "Boring. I can never eat what I like again."

Weight loss is: "Hard. I don't think I can keep it off."

When I lose weight: "I'll get attention, and I don't think I can handle that."

Another reason we sabotage our desire to lose weight, begin an exercise program, or take on any challenge in our life is our fear of living with the fact that you may have let someone down. It could be you. I have witnessed this on many occasions working with student athletes. Whenever they were unsure of their ability, I would ask them, "What would happen if you failed?"

Their response was textbook. "I let everyone down."

This fear has paralyzed many. Is the bigger regret trying something new and failing or never even trying?

Could you be sabotaging your weight loss? Are you dealing with factors other than relying on food for energy?

Remember that food was intended to be used for nourishment and was never intended to be overconsumed or used for fun. Ironically, when we use food for fun, our bodies have no fun at all. Our bodies have to work harder, and over time, they cannot fight off the effects of this mistreatment. The result is that we gain more weight, clog our arteries, and put more strain on our hearts. Hopefully, you could decide that fun is being healthy and happy and changing your entire belief system about food.

Repair and Recovery

What has helped me in selecting the type and quantity of food I consume is the fact that recovery from exercise is an all-day process. In fact, it takes twenty-four to forty-eight hours to fully replace our energy stores. Therefore, I look at every meal as repair and recovery meals. What kind of repair and recovery is going to take place in my body with a bag of chips and a soda?

One of the best ways to add years to your life and life to your years is to eat less, move more, and eat smart foods.

Here are the smart foods I rely on.

- Beet juice. Some endurance athletes drink beet juice based on the belief that it may improve blood and oxygen flow in their muscles during training and competition. Some strength and power athletes consume it with the hopes that it can improve their ability to withstand muscle fatigue during repeated bouts of high-intensity exercise. Although there is no proof it helps with performance, I consume it knowing there are many other health benefits. What's there to lose?

- Low-fat chocolate milk. Several years ago, the NCAA randomly tested products marketed as post-workout recovery drinks. In its testing, it discovered that some products contained trace amounts of steroids, which are illegal and banned by the NCAA. If an athlete tested positive, he or she would lose a scholarship and eligibility to play. To assist the athletes with recovery, the NCAA tested various products. The one that scored the highest was low-fat chocolate milk. It was the perfect combination of protein and carbohydrates to help recover, especially when consumed within thirty to sixty minutes after exercise. This is the time your body is able to synthesize glycogen from the carbohydrates you eat at a much faster rate. Your heart rate and blood pressure also are elevated, so nutrients are delivered to your muscles and cells more quickly.

- Tart cherry juice. Recent studies conclude that Montmorency cherry juice can have an impact on athletic performance and recovery. It has proven to be an effective and functional food for accelerating recovery by reducing exercise-induced inflammation following strenuous exercise. Those with chronic kidney disease need to be careful since overdosing on cherry concentrate could further damage kidneys.

- Vitamins and minerals. There are many pros and cons regarding the need for taking vitamin and mineral supplements. There is a recommended dietary allowance (RDA) that estimates the amount of nutrients per day that are considered necessary for the maintenance of good health. Due to the fact that so much of the food we consume today is processed and that we are not consuming fruit fresh off the vine or meat just butchered like the meals consumed by my boyhood heroes, I take vitamin and mineral supplements daily as an insurance policy that I am getting at least the RDA. The vitamins I consume are made by Shaklee Corporation. One of the reasons I choose Shaklee is that it is one of the few vitamin companies that will guarantee absorbency of their products. Some products are taken and endorsed by Olympic athletes.

A word of caution: Please avoid supplements marketed for weight loss and boosting energy. Many of these products can cause cardiac symptoms such as palpitations, chest pain, and rapid heartbeat and have caused many users to seek medical attention and even to be rushed to the emergency room.

If you decide to take vitamins, be sure to check with your doctor and do your research.

Diet

I never use the word "diet' with my clients. The first three letters spell "die", plus I have discovered that one size does not fit all when using a diet plan. There is no single diet that is right for everyone. Many of the popular low-calorie diets are actually dangerous and slow your metabolism. Your metabolism remains slow, which results in more weight gain when you resume a normal diet.

I prefer mini meals. I will use the term "breakfast" because that is the break after the fast. If you've slept for seven or eight hours, you have fasted. Therefore, your first meal of the day is the perfect opportunity to feed yourself breakfast. You should then consume several mini meals throughout the day. Have you have ever witnessed brand-new babies feeding? They eat and stop and eat and stop many times a day. They are so connected with their feelings of hunger and being satisfied. That is how all of us are designed—to eat and stop, eat and stop—not consume food two or three times a day or to skip meals all day and eat one large one. I calculate the number of meals needed per day as follows. The first thing to do is to calculate my protein requirement. When you exercise you need 0.8 grams of protein per pound of body weight. For example, if I weigh 200 pounds, my daily protein requirement is 160 grams (200 X 0.8). A human can absorb and digest only twenty-four grams of protein at a time. Therefore, my daily protein requirement of 160 grams is divided by twenty-four grams maximum per meal, which means that I should have 6.6 or 7 meals per day.

You may be asking what you should eat.

When you are exercising, you are now an athlete. (I believe all of us are born athletes, but some of us train while some do not.) It's important to look at food and meals as fuel. We need fuel to get us through our workouts and fuel to help us recover for the next workout. It takes us twenty-four to forty-eight hours after a workout to recover, so our meals should consist of carbohydrates (to replace glycogen), protein (to repair muscle and tissue damage caused by the stress of working out), and fluids (for hydration). According to the registered dietitians who advise NCAA athletes, during hard training days, half of our plate should be whole grains or other energy-enhancing foods. A quarter of our plate should be lean protein, and the final quarter of our plate should be fruits and vegetables. On light training days, half of our plate should be fruits and vegetables, one quarter of our plate should be whole grain or other energy-enhancing food, and the final quarter of our plate should be lean protein. Adequate fluids are consumed with meals and throughout the day.

There are 3,500 calories in one pound. If your goal is weight loss, in order to lose one pound a week, you must reduce your daily calories by 500. (500 calories per day X 7 days = 3,500 calories per week). I recommend moving more to burn 500 due to the fact that there are so many more health benefits when we move our bodies than just reducing calories. Exercise not only burns calories, but it also makes you trimmer and fitter and helps prevent loss of muscle mass and the drop in metabolic rate that usually accompanies dieting. Even when you achieve your desired weight, exercise is an effective way to prevent or minimize future weight gain. Our bodies were designed to move. We were meant to move. Where have you heard that before?

CHAPTER 8

TIPS FOR SUCCESS

Over the past twenty years working as a personal trainer, I have discovered a few tips to make your exercise session successful. Besides the fact that you should be properly hydrated, well-rested, and eating the smart foods to enhance performance, I recommend the following tips.

- Check with your doctor. Before you begin any exercise program check with your doctor. The last thing you want to do is cause injury or harm to yourself. The goal is to be healthy.
- Be patient. The most frequent question I hear when someone begins to exercise is when results will become apparent. You must realize that exercise does not work like a microwave oven. You cannot begin and become fit and healthy within minutes. If I had a microscope and looked at your muscle fibers after exercise, we would see immediate changes. Unfortunately, the visual changes you are looking for take time. Many of us have high and unrealistic expectations regarding our appearance because we are bombarded with exercise and diet programs that promote unrealistic results. If you have exercised in the past, stopped (for whatever reason), and resumed again, you would see results quickly. That is my definition of muscle memory. You're muscles remember how to perform. If you are sedentary, there is a process that takes time in which your brain and your muscles have to get in sync. This could take a few months.

Be patient! Like many things in health and life, there is no quick fix.

- Accept your genetics. When it comes to how we look in the mirror, try to avoid comparing yourself to others. You are a product of your mother and father, and there is no one, nor will there ever be another, like you. You are unique and possess unique genetics. Regardless of hereditary, regular exercise, both aerobic and strength training, will result in an improvement in the quality of your life.

- Give your best. Know that your best changes day to day, moment to moment. For example, if you are fighting off a cold, your best will not be the same as if you are in good health. If you didn't get a good night's sleep, your best that day will not be the same as if you got a good eight hours of sleep. Do your best under the circumstances.

- More on sleep. I cannot emphasize how important it is to get at least eight hours of sleep each night. I witness so many people, who due to a lack of sleep, rely on preworkout drinks loaded with sugar and caffeine to get them through their workout and provide energy for daily activities. Poor eating habits, lack of sleep, and other factors that we control have created the multibillion-dollar supplement industry that exists today. Our bodies were designed to function with food, not supplements.

- Think happy thoughts. I have a client who is a grandmother. Whenever she is performing a set of any exercise and the final reps are becoming difficult, I will mention her grandchildren. Her eyes open widely, she gets the biggest grin on her face, and the reps keep coming. I have another client who loves lighthouses, and her hobby is to collect them. When she is starting to fatigue during her set, all I have to do is mention lighthouses, and the results are great.

  In studies of weightlifters, some were told to get mad and angry when lifting while others were told to think about a joyous time in their life. Those who felt a positive emotion lifted more weight and executed more reps.

Along with thinking happy thoughts, another method I use to motivate my clients to get that extra rep is that I avoid the words don't, not, and no. For example, if I told you not to think about a snowstorm or the Statue of Liberty, you would. For some reason, our brains do not process the words don't, not, and no. When applying this principle to exercise, I say exactly what I want from my client. I say, "Stay strong" instead of "Don't quit." Maybe that's why, when I was a young boy and my mother told me not to touch the hot stove, I did. Ouch!

• Set realistic goals. Identify and state your goal then take small steps to achieve it. At the high school where I was the strength and conditioning coach, our boys' basketball team was struggling to win games. The boys were starting to doubt their ability to win. During one of our weight-training sessions, I started the session by sharing one of my observations. "You know," I said, "If you guys score sixty points in a game, you'll win it. I noticed that even the best team in the league is averaging fifty-five points per game."

"How do you expect us to do that?" asked one of the boys.

"Well, you need sixty points to win, which means you'll need thirty points by halftime. Since the game is played in quarters, that means you'll need fifteen points at the end of each quarter. There are five of you guys playing. Do you think it's possible that each of you score three points each quarter? If each of you score three points, that's fifteen points per quarter. Heck, maybe one of you gets hot and scores seven points." Their eyes lit up, they smiled, and they realized they could succeed. Small, achievable steps toward a goal!

• Keep accurate records. To track exercise progress, you should record the weight you used and the reps you executed with that weight. Over time, your muscles will adapt to the resistance used. Then you could challenge yourself by increasing the weight, increasing the reps, or increasing the time under load as long as you adhere to the HIT principles of perfect form, working hard, and using a high level of intensity. If you are in the process of weight loss, the more you track, the more you'll learn about your eating habits, and the more likely you'll be to reach your goals.

- Keep strength training and cardiovascular work separate. When it comes to exercise, we all assume that more is better. I believe that is true if you are practicing a sport skill, such as a basketball player shooting 100 foul shots. Since your muscles grow in size and muscular ability when you rest and recover, it is critical to take a day or two between workouts. I also believe that we should be active every day. Therefore, I recommend doing cardiovascular work on the days off from lifting. Because exercise is the controlled tearing of muscle tissue, in order to control the trauma of working muscles, I recommend sprinting on cardiovascular days. Sprinting gives you the endurance needed to lift weights, and lifting weights gives you the strength needed to run. If you are unable to sprint and enjoy walking, you can mix up your pace. You can walk your comfortable pace, speed it up for a few seconds, slow down for double the speed pace, and repeat. Sprinting is not limited to running or walking. If you cycle, jump rope, use a treadmill, use an elliptical machine, or perform any other cardiovascular activity, you can sprint. The important thing is to get your heart rate up and then down.
- Stretching. There is an ongoing debate over the subject of stretching. To stretch or not to stretch, that is the question. I believe stretching improves your range of motion, protects joints, and improves muscular performance to guard against the low back pain that is very common as we age.
I find stretching extremely relaxing, and many athletes stretch to maintain flexibility and a balance in body mechanics. I recommend it because it feels great. Should you decide to stretch, aim to hold your stretch comfortably for one minute. Relax and breathe!
- Pamper yourself and heal. Along with witnessing HIT training at Penn State, I was amazed at how much attention the athletes received after their training session. After the weight training and running sessions, the athletes spent another hour with the

athletic training department stretching, icing, heating, receiving massage, and whatever other treatment the athlete needed for recovery. Many of us train hard and then go about our daily lives. We never spend any time after our workouts pampering our bodies the way athletes do. I encourage you to take time after your training to pamper and heal. Massage, warm bath, chiropractic care, meditation, stretching, and relaxation are just a few examples of pampering. What's your favorite way to pamper? What would you enjoy?

- Quick and easy nutrition tips. Always stay hydrated, eat for recovery and repair, and stop when you feel full but not stuffed.

- What you believe can be a powerful force regarding sickness and health. Many studies link our health to our emotions. The emotions that can weaken us are fear, envy, anger, resentment, and sorrow. What can strengthen us are faith in God, exercise, acceptance, relaxation, and singing. Both of these are acronyms for FEARS.

CHAPTER 9

SAMPLE EXERCISE PROGRAM

The National Federation of Professional Trainers Study and Reference Manual states that contraindications to all forms of exercise include joint pain, dizziness, nausea, rapid pulse, excessive sweating, extreme muscle soreness, cramping, and chest pain. Upon occurrence of one or more of the above, stop exercising and consult with your physician.

Remember that contraindications to all forms of exercise include joint pain, dizziness, nausea, rapid pulse, excessive sweating, extreme muscle soreness, cramping, and chest pain. Upon occurrence of one or more of the above, stop exercising and consult with your physician.

Day 1

Exercise																
	Date															
Ball Squats	lbs.															
	reps.															
Leg Curl	lbs.															
	reps.															
Ball 1																
	reps.															
Ball 2																
	reps.															
Chest Press	lbs.															
	reps.															
Lat Pulldown	lbs.															
	reps.															
Chest Fly	lbs.															
	reps.															
Low Row	lbs.															
	reps.															
Side Raise	lbs.															
	reps.															
Front Raise	lbs.															
	reps.															
Rear Raise	lbs.															
	reps.															
Tricep Pushdown	lbs.															
	reps.															
Bicep Curl	lbs.															
	reps.															
Abdominals																

Day 2 Cardiovascular

220 - _____ (your age) = _____ your maximum heart rate (MHR)
60% of your maximum heart rate = _____
65% of your maximum heart rate = _____
70% of your maximum heart rate = _____
75% of your maximum heart rate = _____
80% of your maximum heart rate = _____
85% of your maximum heart rate = _____

The Workout

Warm up one minute.

Four forty-second second sprints with eighty seconds (or longer rest) between sprints in order to achieve sixty percent of MHR.

Eight thirty-second sprints with sixty seconds (or longer rest) between sprints in order to achieve sixty percent of MHR.

Ten twenty-second sprints with forty seconds (or longer rest) between sprints to achieve sixty percent of MHR.

I encourage you to get creative with this workout. Your goal is to sprint for a total of ten minutes.

Another example would be as follows.

Two forty-second sprints with eighty seconds (or longer rest) between sprints to achieve sixty percent of MHR.

Eight thirty-second sprints with sixty seconds (or longer rest) between sprints to achieve sixty percent of MHR.

Eight twenty-second sprints with forty seconds (or longer rest) between sprints to achieve sixty percent of MHR.

Eight fifteen-second sprints with thirty seconds (or longer rest) between sprints to achieve sixty percent of MHR.

Remember that contraindications to all forms of exercise include joint pain, dizziness, nausea, rapid pulse, excessive sweating, extreme muscle soreness, cramping, and chest pain. Upon occurrence of one or more of the above, stop exercising and consult with your physician.

Remember that contraindications to all forms of exercise include joint pain, dizziness, nausea, rapid pulse, excessive sweating, extreme muscle soreness, cramping, and chest pain. Upon occurrence of one or more of the above, stop exercising and consult with your physician.

Day 3

Exercise																		
	Date																	
Hip	lbs.																	
Adduction	reps.																	
Hip	lbs.																	
Abduction	reps.																	
Ball 3																		
	reps.																	
Ball 4																		
	reps.																	
Calf Raise	lbs.																	
	reps.																	
Chest Press	lbs.																	
	reps.																	
Lat	lbs.																	
Pushdown	reps.																	
Ball 5																		
	reps.																	
Low Row	lbs.																	
	reps.																	
Tricep	lbs.																	
Pushdown	reps.																	
Bicep Curl	lbs.																	
	reps.																	
Abdominals																		

Day 4 Cardiovascular

The Workout

Warm up one minute.

Ten one-minute sprints with a two-minute (or longer) rest in between sprints to achieve sixty percent of your MHR.

Remember that contraindications to all forms of exercise include joint pain, dizziness, nausea, rapid pulse, excessive sweating, extreme muscle soreness, cramping, and chest pain. Upon occurrence of one or more of the above, stop exercising and consult with your physician.

CHAPTER 10

EXERCISE TIPS AND ILLUSTRATIONS

The sample strength-training exercises are performed on the equipment I have available. The exercise equipment is not important and can vary. What is important is that you apply the following three guidelines.

1. Stop if you if you experience any of the contraindications to exercise: joint pain, dizziness, nausea, rapid pulse, excessive sweating, extreme muscle soreness, cramping, and chest pain. If you experience any of these, consult with your physician.
2. Slowly work all three components of the exercise: the lifting component, the pause under the weight component, and the lowering component.
3. It's not the weight you use. It's how you use the weight.

To select the proper weight (resistance) and proper repetition range, you must identify your personal goal.

Goal	Repetition range
Size and strength	Four to six
Athlete	Eight to twelve
General fitness	Twelve to fifteen
Weight loss/endurance	Twenty to twenty-five

For example, if your personal goal is general fitness, select a weight (resistance) that will allow you to perform twelve to fifteen repetitions slowly while pausing under the weight (resistance) in perfect form through the entire range of motion of the working muscle. If you can perform fewer than twelve repetitions, reduce the weight (resistance). If you can perform fifteen or more repetitions, slightly increase the weight (resistance). This applies to all repetition ranges. Always focus on working your muscle instead of just doing repetitions.

The exercise equipment you choose is not important. The descriptions can be applied to any piece of exercise equipment.

Exercise for the Front of the Leg

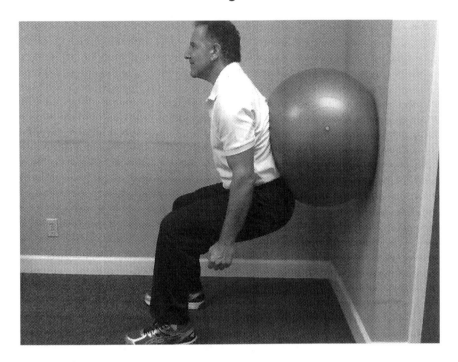

Feet shoulder-width or a little wider apart. Focus forward.

Lowering component: Bend knees and slowly descend. Reach back with your hips as if you are reaching back to sit in a chair. Descend until your thighs are parallel (or higher based on your flexibility) to the floor. Be sure your knees are behind or in alignment with your toes. Keep your heels on the floor.

Pause component: Hold for a count of two.

Lifting component: Slowly come back up, keeping your knees unlocked at the top, and repeat without resting until you cannot perform another repetition in perfect form through the entire muscle range of motion.

Exercise for the Back of the Leg

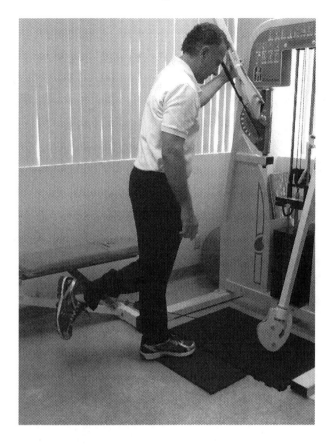

Lifting component: Slowly curl the leg (or legs if you are using a seated or lying leg curl machine) toward the buttocks as far as you can without engaging your hips.

Pause component: Hold for a count of two.

Lowering component: Slowly lower the leg (or legs) to the starting position and repeat without resting until you cannot perform another repetition in perfect form through the entire muscle range of motion.

Exercise for the Hips

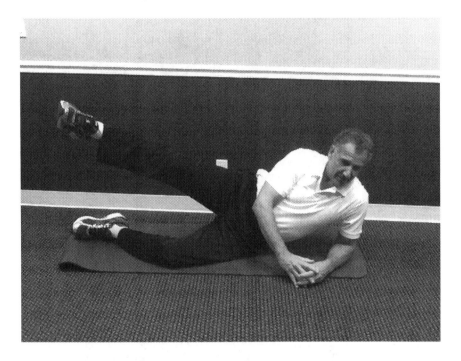

Abduction (moving legs away from the center of your body).

Lifting component: Slowly lift (or push if you are using an abduction machine) your leg (or legs) away from the midline of your body without any twisting or jerking.

Pause component: Hold for a count of two.

Lowering component: Slowly bring your leg (or legs) back to the starting position and repeat without resting in the starting position until you cannot perform another repetition in perfect form through the entire muscle range of motion.

Exercise for the Inner Thigh

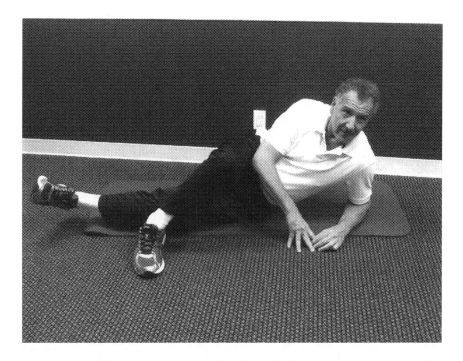

Adduction (moving your legs toward the center of your body).

Lifting component: Slowly lift (or push if you are using an adduction machine) your leg (or legs) toward the midline of your body without any twisting or jerking.

Pause component: Hold for a count of two.

Lowering component: Slowly bring your leg (or legs) back to the starting position and repeat without resting in the starting position until you cannot perform another repetition in perfect form through the entire muscle range of motion.

Exercise for the Lower Leg

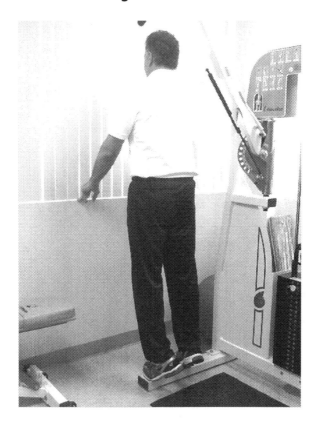

Lifting component: Slowly rise up as high as possible on your toes without bending your knees for assistance.

Pause component: Hold for a count of two.

Lowering component: Slowly lower your heels as low as possible repeat without resting until you cannot perform another repetition in perfect form through the entire muscle range of motion.

Exercises for the Core

I recommend performing exercises for your core using a stability ball (often referred to as a Swiss, exercise, or physio ball). When you are performing movements on the ball, the ball wants to roll. You must control the ball using the muscles of your core while executing the movement. They are inexpensive, challenging, and effective for training your core.

Be sure to use a stability ball that is the proper diameter for your height.

Ball diameter	User height
45 cm	4'6" to 5'0"
55 cm	5'1" to 5'7"
65 cm	5'8" to 6'1"
75 cm	6'2" to 6'7"

Movement 1

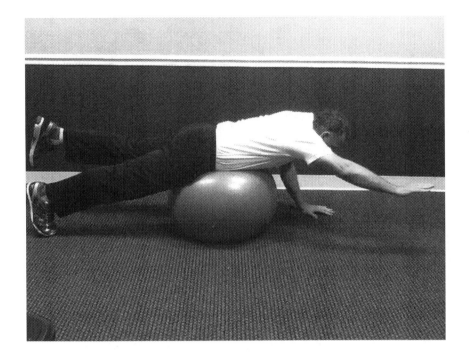

Begin face down, and keep your arms and legs straight.

Lifting component. Slowly lift an opposite arm and opposite leg at the same time without bending your knees or elbows. Lift as if someone is stretching you at the wrist and ankle.

Pause component. Hold for a count of two as if someone is taking your picture (smile).

Lowering component. Slowly lower your arm and leg at the same time and repeat without rest. After completing repetitions until you cannot perform another repetition in perfect form through the entire muscle range of motion, switch to the opposite arm and leg.

To add difficulty to this exercise, perform the exercise with your hand off the floor and resting on the ball or your lower back.

Movement 2

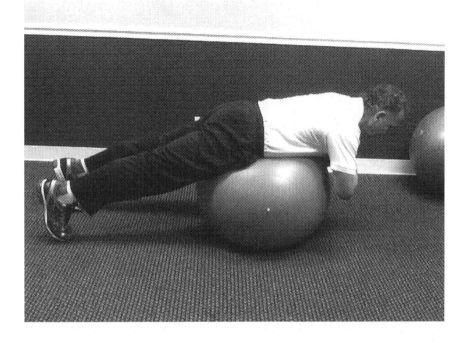

Lifting component: Using your lower back strength, slowly lift your upper body.

Pause component: Hold for a count of two.

Lowering component: Slowly lower yourself and repeat without rest until you cannot perform another repetition in perfect form through the entire muscle range of motion.

Movement 3

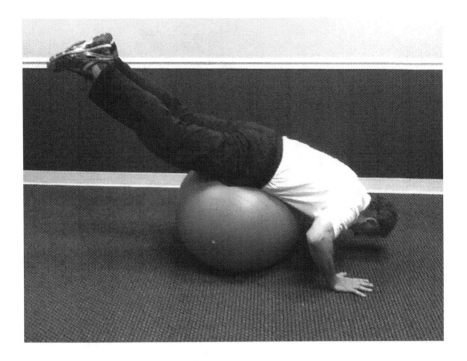

Begin face down with your elbows bent so that your face is a few inches from the floor.

Lifting component: Using your lower back strength, slowly lift your legs.

Pause component: Hold for a count of two.

Lowering component: Slowly lower your legs and repeat without rest until you cannot perform another repetition in perfect form through the entire muscle range of motion.

Movement 4

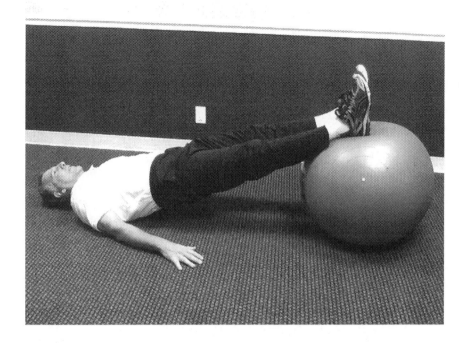

Lie on your back and rest your legs on the ball.

Lifting component: Slowly lift your buttocks a small distance from the floor and squeeze your buttocks tight.

Pause component: Squeeze for a count of two.

Lowering component: Slowly lower your buttocks and repeat without rest until you cannot perform another repetition in perfect form through the entire muscle range of motion.

Movement 5

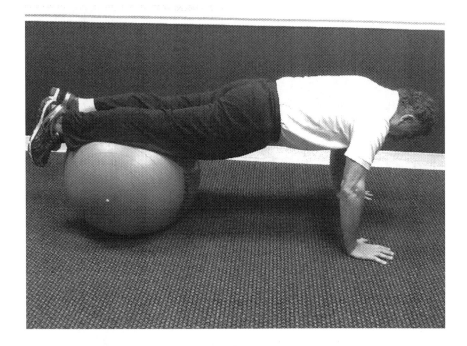

Begin face down with hands in a push-up position.

Lifting component: Slowly walk out using your arm strength without sagging your hips to the floor.

Pause component: Hold for a count of two.

Lowering component: Slowly return to the starting position and repeat without rest until you cannot perform another repetition in perfect form through the entire muscle range of motion.

To add difficulty to this exercise, perform the pause component of the exercise with just your toes on the ball.

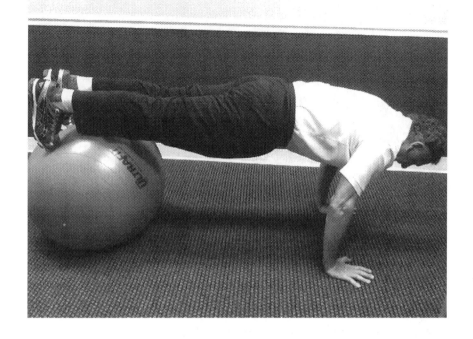

Exercises for the Upper Body

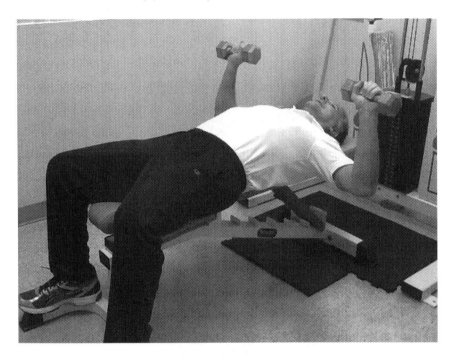

Chest press: Lie on a flat bench or an incline bench or sit upright on a chest press machine.

Lowering component: Breathe in and slowly lower the weight to your chest, stopping just short of your chest.

Pause component: Hold for a count of two.

Lifting component: Breathe out and slowly push the weight up until your elbows are soft. Repeat without rest until you cannot perform another repetition in perfect form through the entire muscle range of motion.

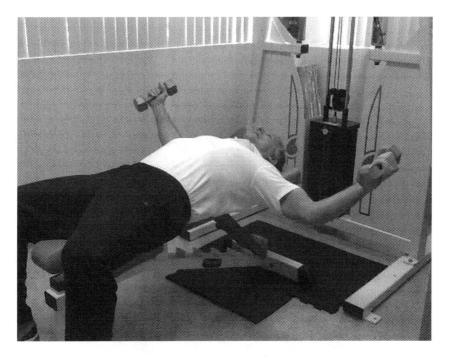

Chest fly: Lie on a flat bench or an incline bench or sit upright on a chest fly machine.

Lowering component: Breathe in and slowly lower the weight out to the side of your chest until a comfortable stretch is felt across your chest and the front of your shoulders.

Pause component: Hold for a count of two.

Lifting component: Breathe out and slowly bring the weight back to the midpoint of your chest in the same path you used for the lowering component. (Imagine that you are hugging a big tree.) Repeat without rest until you cannot perform another repetition in perfect form through the entire muscle range of motion.

Exercises for the Back

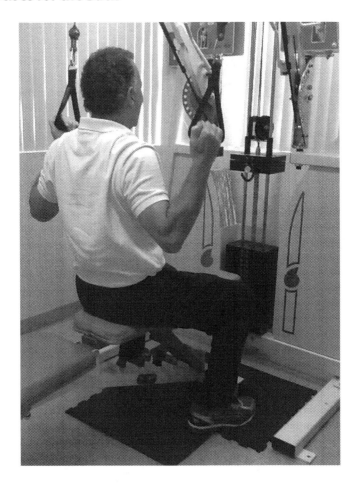

Lat pulldown: This exercise requires a lat pulldown machine. Regardless of whether you use a bar or individual handles, sit upright facing the machine with your thighs secured under the pad (if there is one). Grip the bar (handles) with your palms facing you. I recommend not using your thumbs when you grip. Your hands are just connectors to the bar (handles).

Lifting component: Slowly pull the bar (handles) down to just above the chest as if you want to drive your elbows into your back pocket. Avoid using your arms to pull and relax your grip.

Pause component: Maintain a neutral back and squeeze your shoulder blades together for a count of two. Maintain an upright posture, and avoid leaning back throughout the exercise.

Lowering component: Slowly raise the weight back to the starting position. Repeat without rest until you cannot perform another repetition in perfect form through the entire muscle range of motion.

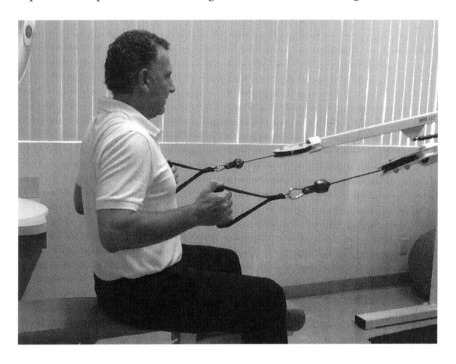

Low row: This exercise requires a seated row machine or low cable pulley. Grasp the handles with your palms facing each other. I recommend not using our thumbs when you grip. Your hands are just connectors to the handles. Start with your arms fully extended.

Lifting component: Slowly pull the handles straight back, squeezing your shoulder blades together. Avoid using your arms to pull and relax your grip. Your elbows should lightly brush by your sides.

Frank Manganella

Pause component: Hold for a count of two. Maintain a tall posture throughout the exercise, and avoid leaning back or toward the machine with your head.

Lowering component: Slowly return to the starting position, and repeat without rest until you cannot perform another repetition in perfect form through the entire muscle range of motion.

Exercises for the Shoulders

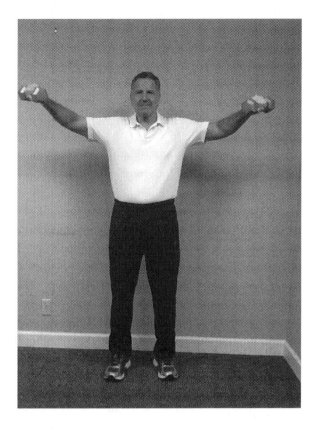

Side lateral raise (fly like a bird): Stand with your feet shoulder-width apart and knees slightly bent. Maintain a straight back.

Lifting component: With palms facing each other and elbows slightly bent, slowly raise your arms out to the side until elbows are at shoulder height.

Pause component: Hold for a count of two. Keep your elbows slightly bent throughout the exercise and relax your grip.

Lowering component: Slowly lower your arms to the starting position, and repeat without rest until you cannot perform another repetition in perfect form through the entire muscle range of motion. This exercise is just like a bird slowly flying.

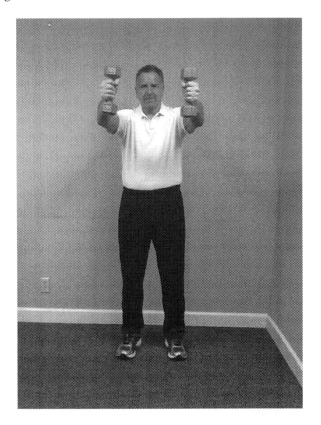

Front raise (baby wearing a stinky diaper): Stand with your feet shoulder-width apart and knees slightly bent throughout the exercise.

Lifting component: Slowly raise your arms in front of you (as if you were handing someone a baby who is wearing a smelly diaper). Keep your arms parallel to the floor.

Pause component: Hold for a count of two. Keep your elbows slightly bent throughout the exercise, and relax your grip.

Lowering component: Slowly lower your arms to the starting position, and repeat without rest until you cannot perform another repetition in perfect form through the entire muscle range of motion.

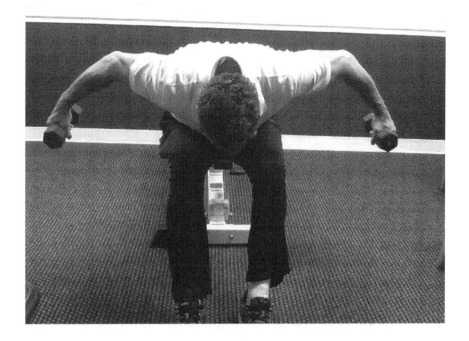

Rear raise: Lean forward so that your torso rests on your thighs, palms facing each other.

Lifting component: Keeping your elbows slightly bent, and slowly raise your arms to the side.

Pause component: Hold for a count of two. Keep your elbows slightly bent throughout the exercise, and relax your grip.

Lowering component: Slowly lower your arms to the starting position, and repeat without rest until you cannot perform another repetition in perfect form through the entire muscle range of motion.

Exercises for the Arms

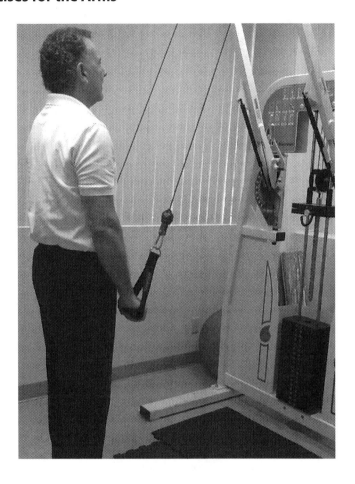

Triceps pushdown: A high pulley cable is needed for this exercise. Stand straight up with a soft bend in your knees. Flex your elbows while grasping the cable attachment without using your thumbs.

Lifting component: Slowly extend your arms down and push toward the floor until your elbows are just shy of locking. Keep your neck and lower back in a neutral position.

Pause component: Hold for a count of two.

Lowering component: Slowly bend your elbows to the starting position, and repeat without rest until you cannot perform another repetition in perfect form through the entire muscle range of motion.

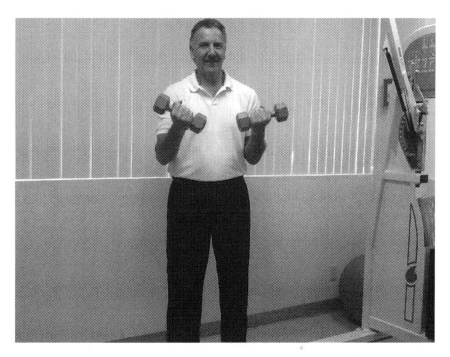

Bicep curl: Grasp the weight (resistance) with your palms facing away from your body.

Lifting component: Slowly bend your elbows and pull your arms up to where your elbows are bent at 130 degrees.

Pause component: Hold for a count of two. Keep your grip soft, and if you are standing, avoid rocking forward and backward at your hips.

Lowering component: Slowly lower your arms to the starting position, and repeat without rest until you cannot perform another repetition in perfect form through the entire muscle range of motion.

Exercises for the Abdominals

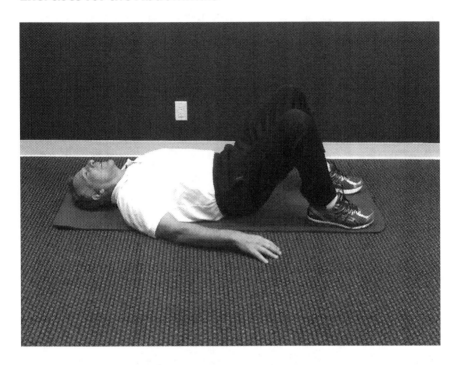

Pelvic tilt one: Lying face up with your knees bent, push your lower back into the floor. This should cause you to roll your hips up toward your head. You could also imagine someone dropping a heavy bowling ball on your stomach. Hold your back flat on the floor for a count of three, release, and repeat for twelve repetitions.

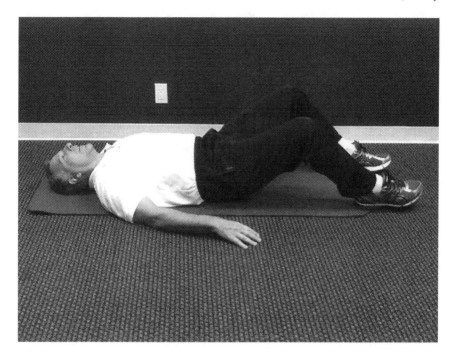

Pelvic tilt two: This is the same as pelvic tilt one, but move your feet farther away from your body.

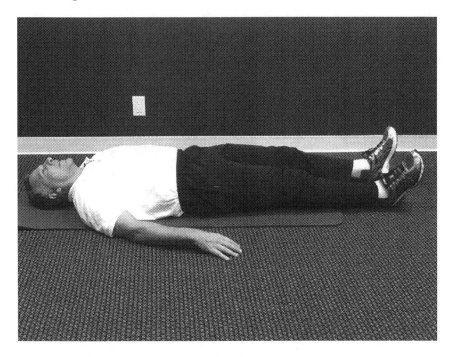

Pelvic tilt three: This is the same as pelvic tilt one, except that you are now lying flat.

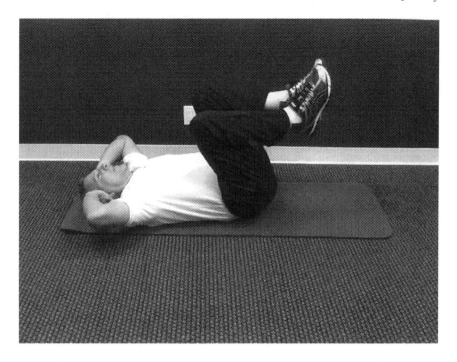

Knees to your chest: Lying face up with your knees bent, bring bent knees of the floor

Lifting component: Pull you knees close enough to your chest so that your back is flat. This is the starting position. Using your lower abdominal strength to slowly bring your knees closer to your chest.

Pause component: Hold for a count of two.

Lowering component: Slowly return to the starting position, and repeat for twelve repetitions.

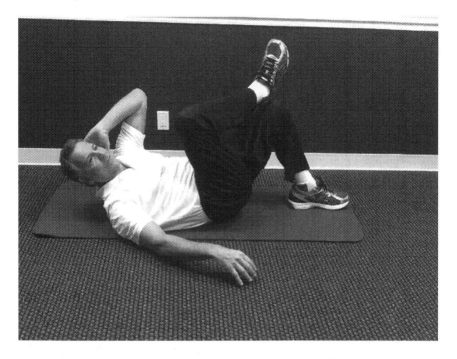

Opposite elbow to knee crunch: Lying face up with your knees bent, bring one leg up and rest your ankle on your knee. Place the opposite hand behind your ear, and rest it softly.

Lifting component: Tilt your pelvis, and slowly pull your trunk up and twist without putting any pressure on the back of your neck.

Pause component: Hold for a count of two.

Lowering component: Slowly return to the starting position, and repeat for twelve repetitions.

To add difficulty to this exercise, at the pause component of the twelfth repetition, pulse for twelve additional repetitions.

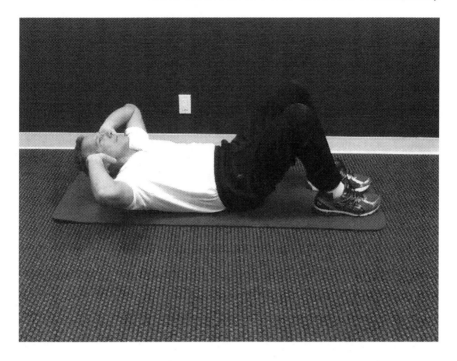

Crunch: Lying face up with your knees bent, place your hands in the following positions based on your level of experience:

Beginner: Hands reaching to the ceiling.

Intermediate: Hands resting on your chest.

Advanced: Hands placed softly behind your ears.

Elite: Arms extended straight behind your head.

Lifting component: Tilt your pelvis, and slowly raise your head, shoulders, and scapulae off the floor without reaching with your neck.

Pause component: Hold for a count of two.

Lowering component: Slowly return to the starting position, and repeat for twelve repetitions.

CHAPTER 11

WHAT TO DO IF YOU ARE NEW TO EXERCISE

You've decided or have been advised by your doctor to start weight training. You drive to your local fitness center, park your car, and observe all the people entering and leaving. You get cold feet. Something inside you tells you that you can't do this. You feel intimidated and find yourself driving back home.

Fitness centers and gyms can make you feel anxious and overwhelmed. You see people and machines everywhere. Everybody seems to know what they are doing. Some could be working with a trainer, while others may be in a separate room (or rooms) taking classes. I would like to help ease your anxiety and give you a few tips.

One, visit the fitness center or gym at a time when you will be using it.

This will enable you to see just how crowded and busy it is, who is working the front desk, and whether there is equipment available for you to use. Feel the energy in the facility. Are you comfortable, or is something not right? We are very intuitive. Use your intuition to your advantage. If you feel comfortable, proceed to the next tip.

Two, ask for a tour of the facility. Say you are interested in weight training, and try to keep the tour in that area of the facility. I recommend you ask to see the following:

- Equipment to perform your warmups and sprinting. Treadmills, stationary bikes, and elliptical trainers are excellent pieces.

Which piece feels right to you, and is it available for you to use at this time of day?

- An area for stretching, an area for stability ball exercises, and an area for you to perform your abdominal exercises.
- Are there any stability balls? If so, how many can you choose from for your specific height?
- Equipment for you to perform your strength training. I'm sure you will see numerous machines with cables and pulleys, many weights, bars, dumbbells, hanging straps, kettlebells, ropes, and more. Following the days one and three workouts in this book, have the person giving the tour show you the various equipment that you could use starting with exercising the front of your legs. Ask for a demonstration of how to use it. Many pieces have seat adjustments and/or back adjustments, and you want to make sure the adjustments are correct for your specific height. After you witness the demonstration, give it a try. Does this piece of equipment feel right to you? Listen to your intuition. Is the equipment available for you to use at this time of the day? Proceed to the various equipment for exercising the backs of your legs, the equipment for exercising your hips, and so on. At each piece of equipment, ask for a demonstration, check to see if the piece has seat and/or back adjustments, and see what the proper settings for your height are. Give it a try. Is it available for you to use at this time of day? Choose the piece of equipment that feels right. The piece of equipment is not important. Rather, how you use the equipment is important. The various pieces of equipment offer you options to perform the exercise movements described in this book.

You should feel very comfortable and able to perform your exercise program. When you start exercising, be sure to keep in mind the contradictions to all forms of exercise listed elsewhere in this book.

For executing the sprinting program as described on days two and four, I highly recommend that you purchase an inexpensive heart rate monitor. Usually, it comes with a transmitter that you wear across your chest and a receiver that may look like a wristwatch. This will allow you to accurately monitor your exercising and resting heart rate. Remember to always take enough time between sprints to allow your heart rate to return to sixty percent of maximum. Over time, you will see your conditioning improve. It's exciting when you can actually see your heart getting stronger.

ONE FINAL MESSAGE

I spent two years studying reiki, a form of spiritual healing founded in Japan. In my studies, I discovered a very powerful teaching that always helps me whenever I feel emotions that weaken me.

Just for Today: Five Spiritual Principles of Reiki

Just for today

    I shall trust

Just for today

    I shall do my work honestly

Just for today

    I shall accept my many blessings

Just for today

    I shall be at peace

Just for today

    I will respect the rights of all life forms

Remember, if you want to see your health in the future, look at your lifestyle today. The way you live your life now has a direct effect on your future. You are the architect of your life. You choose to be healthy and fit or sick and frail.

I hope something you read in my book will motivate you to begin exercising. The benefits are numerous.

Find an activity that you find fun and enjoyable that renews and invigorates you. Then stick with it. You will be so happy you did.

Success comes from what you do when no one is looking.

Now that you're convinced that exercise is a good thing, I'm sure you'll find the humor in the following jokes regarding exercise. I know I did.

Exercising can add years to your life. For example, I jogged four miles today, and now I feel like I'm seventy-three.

There are three signs of old age. The first is your loss of memory. The other two I forget.

Walking can add minutes to your life. This enables you to spend an additional five months in a nursing home at $6,000 per month when you are eighty-five.

My grandpa started walking five miles a day when he was sixty. Now he's ninety-seven years old, and we have no idea where the hell he is.

I like long walks, especially when they are taken by people who annoy me.

The only reason I would take up walking is so that I could hear heavy breathing again.

I have to walk early in the morning, before my brain figures out what I'm doing.

I joined a health club last year and spent about $250. Haven't lost a pound. Apparently, you have to go there.

Every time I hear the dirty word "exercise," I wash my mouth out with chocolate.

I do have flabby thighs, but fortunately, my stomach covers them.

The advantage of exercising every day is so that when you die, they'll say,

"Well, he looks good, doesn't he?"

If you are going to try cross-country skiing, start with a small country.

I know I got a lot of exercise the last few years just getting over the hill.

I don't have abs. I have flabs.

To reduce stress, I do yoga. Just kidding, I drink wine in my yoga pants.

We all get heavier as we get older because there's a lot more information in our heads. That's my story, and I'm sticking to it.

Exercise for people over sixty. Begin by standing on a comfortable surface where you have plenty of room at each side. With a five-pound potato bag in each hand, extend your arms straight out from your sides, and hold them there as long as you can. Try to reach a full minute and then relax. Each day, you'll find that you can hold this position for just a bit longer. After a couple of weeks, move up to ten-pound potato bags. Try fifty-pound potato bags, and eventually, try to get to where you can lift a 100-lb potato bag in each hand and hold your arms straight for more than a full minute. (I'm at this level). After you feel confident at that level, put a potato in each bag.

ACKNOWLEDGMENTS

This book came into being because I was encouraged by many clients to tell my story and share my experience as a personal trainer and strength and conditioning coach.

To Allison and Frankie, thank you for understanding my passion for what I do and your patience with me. I am so blessed to have you as my children. I love you.

Thank you, Jeanne Leckey, for your encouragement and participation in this book. The hours you spent reading and rereading, correcting grammar, and assisting with the creation of this book are so greatly appreciated.

Thank you, Mary Wallace. Without your inspiration, my dream of one day writing a book would have never happened. I am so grateful.

Thank you, Emily and Adam Leckey, for the time and effort you put into the photographs and exercise descriptions. I appreciate all the work you both have done.

Thank you, Lauren French, for your excellent photography. Your make me look darn good in those pictures.

Thank you, Jerry Arnese, for believing in my ability and allowing me the opportunity to train your sons, Michael and Jerry.

To Michael Arnese, my first client, and the person responsible for allowing me to find my passion, thank you so much. Without you, none of this was possible.

I cannot begin to put into words my gratitude to John Thomas. You changed my life. You are responsible for me being the man I am.

Your friendship means the world to me. I consider you my mentor and my dearest friend.

Thank you, Jeremy Scott, for teaching me speed development and strength and conditioning. Along with JT, you have had the most impact on my life, and I am so grateful.

Thank you, Mary Ann, for your suggestions, wisdom, and encouragement.

Thank you, Glen Hughes, for your friendship. I am very proud of you.

To the undefeated Bishop Hannan High School freshmen basketball team of 2001–2002, thank you for your hard work and dedication in the weight room. Man! You guys were strong and talented.

To my clients from my gym in Carbondale, Pennsylvania, and the student athletes I had the privilege of training, I cannot thank you enough for your dedication and the effort you put into exercising. I miss all of you.

To the Lakeland Chiefs, thank you to the members of the school board for allowing me the honor of training your student athletes. Thank you to the athletes for your commitment, hard work, and dedication. I had an amazing time. "Set the tone."

To my current clients, you are all amazing. I can't begin to tell you how much I enjoy and look forward to our training sessions. You all work so hard. You all inspire me. Thank you for making me a part of your life. I appreciate and am grateful for each one of you.

ABOUT THE AUTHOR

Frank Manganella is a certified personal trainer with over twenty years of experience. He has successfully trained and coached people of all ages helping them achieve their specific fitness goal. Born in Mayfield, Pennsylvania, he currently resides in Jupiter, Florida.

Printed in the United States
By Bookmasters